Sexuality and learning disability

A guide to supporting continuing professional development

by Zarine Katrak and
Claire Fanstone

First edition published 2003 by FPA

Second edition published by
FPA
50 Featherstone Street
London EC1Y 8QU
Tel: 020 7608 5240
Fax: 0845 123 2349
www.fpa.org.uk

The Family Planning Association is a registered charity, number 250187, and a limited liability company registered in England, number 887632.

© FPA 2011

Printed by Newnorth.

Crown copyright material is reproduced under the terms of the Click-Use Licence.

ISBN: 978-1-905506-82-8

This book can only give you basic information about contraception and sexual health. The information is based on evidence-guided research from the World Health Organization and The Faculty of Sexual and Reproductive Healthcare of the Royal College of Obstetricians and Gynaecologists available at the time this book was printed. Different people may give you different information and advice on certain points. All methods of contraception come with a Patient Information Leaflet which provides detailed information about the method.

Remember – contact your doctor, practice nurse or a contraception or sexual health clinic if you are worried or unsure about anything.

Contents

        page

Acknowledgements 4

About this book 5

Section 1   Introduction – Sexuality work in context 7

Section 2   Sexuality 13

Section 3   Laws, rights and responsibilities 21

Section 4   Policy development 28

Section 5   Spheres of influence 46

Section 6   Skills 60

Section 7   Conclusion 72

Section 8   Useful resources 74

Section 9   Useful organisations 77

Acknowledgements

Many thanks to Denise Souter, Greg Clare, Jim Fagan, Paul Hancock, Mary Thomas, Pat Jackson, Tim Plant, Karen Harms, Helen Peters, Rob Brown, Rachel Pike, Julian Hallett, Victoria Ralfs, Helen Larder, Christine Mortimer, Lauren Mackay, Rachel Davies, Jim Thomas and Sandy Hunt.

About this book

The law in this book relates to England and Wales only. Law in Scotland and Northern Ireland differs to this.

The first edition of this book was published in 2003. It highlighted the legal and policy context for working on diverse issues relating to sexuality with people with learning disabilities. It also captured the dilemmas, insights, positive practice and recommendations of over 200 professionals and carers attending the Learning Disabilities Roadshow.

The Learning Disabilities Roadshow project was managed and run by FPA and offered introductory level training around England. It provided opportunities for multidisciplinary staff and carers to reflect and comment on their professional development needs in this area. The findings of this project became a central part of the 2003 book. It helped to create a practical resource for developing strategies in effective policy, practice and participation underpinning this important area of work.

What is the purpose of this book?

This second edition builds on the first by updating the legal and policy context, retaining relevant issues and adding activities to enable staff and carers to reflect on and inform their practice within the workplace. It also includes a series of checklists and reflections to enable staff to consider how to improve confidence in service delivery when working on issues associated with sexuality for groups and individuals with learning disabilities.

Who is this resource for?

This is a multidisciplinary resource for any staff working with people with learning disabilities to help them reflect on and develop their practice in sexuality work.

A note about terminology in this book

Learning disability
We use this term throughout the publication and acknowledge that there are variations of this term in different areas of the UK.

Person/people with learning disabilities
This is a term we have chosen to use to describe the people you work with or care for who have learning disabilities. In this context it is used in respect of someone who accesses a service and not someone who is dependent on that service.

Parent
The term parent refers to biological parents or foster carers, or the adoptive parents of an individual.

Carer
The term carer refers to anyone caring for a person with a learning disability in a non-professional setting who is not their biological, foster or adoptive parent.

Staff
This term covers a range of professionals, including care workers, community nurses, social services staff, speech and language therapists, health promotion specialists, school nurses, and support staff and their managers, who work with people with learning disabilities.

Introduction – Sexuality work in context

Since the first edition of this book was published, the UK has developed a much stronger culture of inclusion, anti-discrimination and valuing diversity within its laws, policies and duties. For people with learning disabilities in England, local learning disability partnership boards have been guiding the process of inclusion. For many young people and adults with learning disabilities, this has had a positive effect on their personal development, relationships, education and access to a range of services as it supports their individual life choices.

For many other young people and adults with learning disabilities, these benefits have not yet found their way into local policies, guidelines and practice. As a consequence, their ability to exercise their rights and entitlements may be weaker. There has also been an increased reporting of hate crimes to the Home Office in the UK against people with learning disabilities.[1]

> "People with learning difficulties are different to other people. We get picked on – others make fun of us. People shout in the street sometimes. Black people with learning

---

[1] Inclusion North and Coast2Coast, *Learning Disability Hate Crime, Good Practice Guidance for Crime and Disorder Reduction Partnerships and Learning Disability Partnership Boards* (Home Office, 2008).

difficulties get picked on even more. People with learning difficulties should be treated fairly and not discriminated against. Scientists should find the gene that makes people pick on those who are different. Then our lives would be better." [2]

This updated edition of *Sexuality and learning disabilities* explores how staff and carers can uphold entitlements and rights to support individuals to feel safe and empowered to make informed and appropriate choices about their lives.

The case for sexuality work

Despite a strong and positive lead from government via legislation and policy, many people with learning disabilities are still denied their basic human rights by being devalued, discriminated against and abused.

To deny that a person with a learning disability is a sexual being is to devalue them as a person. Avoiding sexuality work can contribute to the discrimination that people with learning disabilities face. This is an ethical and a professional practice issue.

What is sexuality work?

Sexuality work covers the broad areas of sexual health, sex and relationships education (SRE), sexual activity/behaviours, sexual orientation and gender identities; as well as exploring a range of relationships, emotions and self-esteem. It aims to empower people to develop personal and social skills that can foster constructive attitudes and behaviours towards sexual health and wellbeing.

---

[2] Blackman N, *Loss and Learning Disability* (Worth Publishing, 2003).

Why is sexuality work so important for people with learning disabilities?

Upholding the rights of individuals to fairness and freedom, regardless of the issue of learning disability, is a fundamental reason for proactive sexuality work. This rights-based approach is balanced with safety for the individual in living their life.

If people with learning disabilities are unable to recognise what is non-consensual or abusive behaviour and, because of this are unaware of their right to signal (verbally or otherwise) "no", they are at greater risk of being sexually abused.

Preventing abuse and protecting vulnerable adults is an important aspect of delivering effective sexuality work. If issues of abuse are addressed openly and as early as possible with children and young people who have been abused it can increase their personal awareness and responsibility. It can also reduce the potential risk of them progressing from victim to abuser.

Sexuality work is often avoided because of fear. It relates to real concerns that vulnerable people will be sexually exploited or abused and the belief that avoiding all mention of sex and relationships will somehow protect individuals from their sexuality, thus keeping them safe.

Sexuality work is not an optional add on – it is fundamental to the development of identity for any individual with or without a learning disability.

In clarifying what is meant by sexuality work and emphasising the duty of care attached to its delivery, for example in upholding human rights to education and choice, it is possible to allay staff and carers' fears. The benefits of proactive sexuality work can counteract many concerns about vulnerability to abuse and protecting people with learning disabilities by safely promoting their fundamental human rights.

Some staff and carers can find sexuality work embarrassing so it is essential that they find ways of exploring difficult issues such as appropriate public and private behaviour including shows of affection, masturbation or seeking consent in relationships.

With structured reflection and training, issues such as lack of awareness and the inappropriate influence of personal attitudes and beliefs on practice can be addressed. Staff and carers can develop confidence by gaining knowledge and developing skills, awareness and strategies to enable people with learning disabilities to understand and enjoy their rights and the law.

> "I have learnt that people with learning disabilities are not dissimilar to those without, but simply have different issues that are often imposed upon them due to circumstance – not as daunting as I at first thought!"
> **FPA Learning Disabilities Roadshow participant**

Sexuality work – An initial reflection sheet for staff and carers

The worker as a resource

The most important resources for effective sexuality work are skilled, supported and well-trained staff and carers. Reflecting on practice and attending training provides opportunities for staff and carers to identify their professional needs and build their knowledge, skills, awareness and understanding. This will in turn enable staff and carers to feel more confident and competent in delivering sexuality work for people with learning disabilities.

When working with people with learning disabilities on issues of sexuality, how would you assess your knowledge, skills, awareness and understanding? Reflect on each point in the worksheet below and score yourself by asking the following two questions for each point in the grid. Use a scale of 1–5, where **1 = low** and **5 = high**.

1. How **competent (C)** do I feel about this point?

2. How far do I **include (I)** this point in my work currently?

When you have completed the scoring think about what actions you might take to improve your lower scores while valuing the positive aspects of your practice. It might also be useful to discuss your findings with colleagues/other carers and your line manager/supervisor.

1 How would I rate my knowledge about …	C	I	Actions I might like to take
The law?			
The meaning of consent – who can and cannot give it?			
Maintaining professional boundaries?			
Rights and responsibilities of people with learning disabilities, carers and staff?			
National and local policy as well as guidance?			
What constitutes abuse, for example if teaching about masturbation?			
Contraception, sexually transmitted infections and safer sex?			

2 How would I rate my skills in …	C	I	Actions I might like to take
Talking about sex, relationships, sexuality and sexual health?			
Delivering more proactive sexuality work?			
Communicating about the importance of this work to people with learning disabilities, their carers, and colleagues?			
Recognising and getting training and support needs met?			

3 How would I rate my awareness and understanding of …	C	I	Actions I might like to take
Personal values, beliefs and attitudes about sexuality?			
A range of perspectives about all aspects of sexuality?			
Concerns about balancing protection and rights for people with learning disabilities?			
Feelings associated with discrimination experienced by people with learning disabilities?			

Having assessed where you feel you are, the next sections expand on some of the issues that may have arisen for you in completing this worksheet.

Sexuality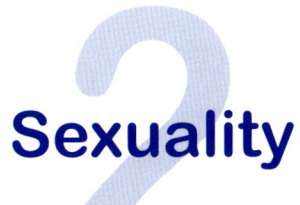

> "Sexuality is a central aspect of being human throughout life and encompasses sex, gender identities and roles, sexual orientation, eroticism, pleasure, intimacy and reproduction. Sexuality is experienced and expressed in thoughts, fantasies, desires, beliefs, attitudes, values, behaviours, practices, roles and relationships. While sexuality can include all of these dimensions, not all of them are always experienced or expressed. Sexuality is influenced by the interaction of biological, psychological, social, economic, political, cultural, ethical, legal, historical, religious and spiritual factors."[3]

Sexuality is an area of life that is fundamental to all people and is expressed every day through beliefs, perception of self, and actions and communication with others. It is important to clarify what sexuality means when working with people with learning disabilities to reduce misunderstandings that lead to staff and carers opposing this area of work. Fear may be at the root of this opposition. This could be based on concerns about exposing those they work with and care for to exploitation and abuse by discussing sexual behaviours.

---

3 World Health Organization, *Defining Sexual Health. Report of a Technical Consultation on Sexual Health 28–31 January 2002* (World Health Organization, 2006).

If sexuality is seen to encompass the spiritual, political, emotional, physical (including the sensual) and intellectual dimensions of a person's identity then fears can be dissipated by the holistic focus of this work.[4]

For staff and carers it is important to discuss and formulate a working definition of sexuality in order to provide a clear structure for doing this work and what influences it. The following key words were among many identified during FPA training courses.

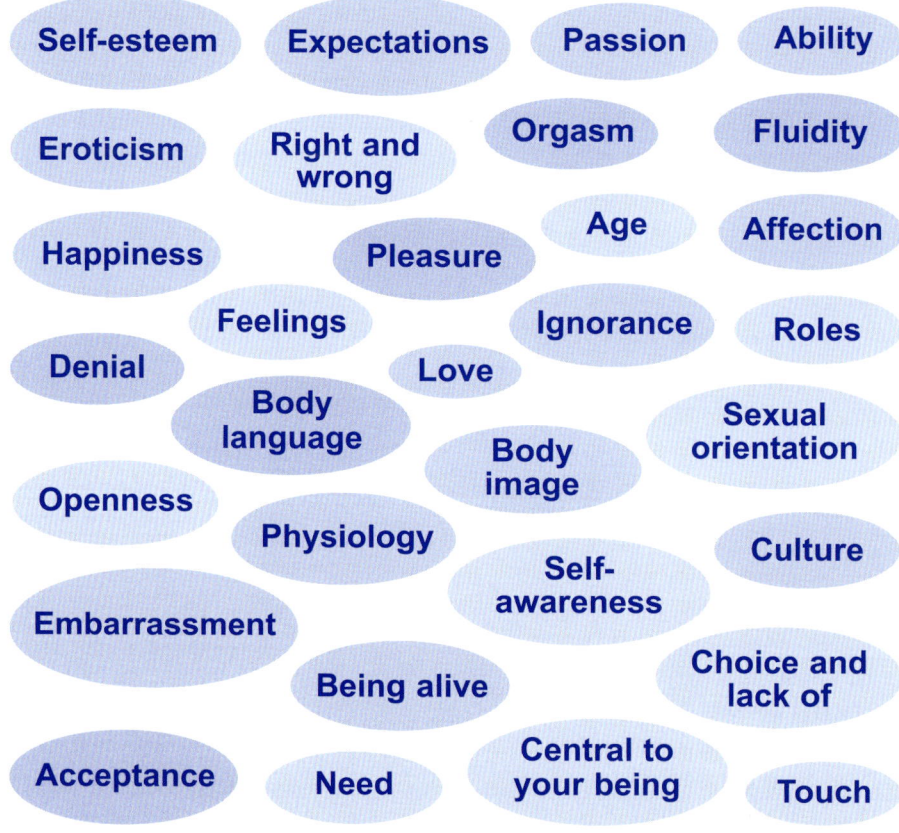

4 Adams J, *Explore, Dream, Discover: Working with Holistic Models of Sexual Health and Sexuality, Self Esteem and Mental Health* (Centre for HIV and Sexual Health, 2005).

Sexuality is...

- **...an outward expression of sensual being and feelings**, governed by both innate and environmental influences which is projected in personality and behaviour

- **...freedom to express individuality** which defines essence, gender and personality

- **...an evolving and changing expression of self-identity** to sustain or gain emotional and physical wellbeing through projection of self to others and their acceptance of your self

- **...a developing process throughout life of expressing your own identity**, your SELF, through your attitudes and the attitudes of others

- **...an expression of self, to self and others**, which is influenced by a combination of biological instinct, cultural and personal experiences and psychological development which changes and progresses through life

- **...a personal expression of an individual's masculinity or femininity** based on behaviour, lifestyle choices, experiences and the way they choose to present themselves in society

- **...an individual's right to be able to express themselves** spiritually, physically, intellectually, emotionally and socially without fear or prejudice

- **...a lifelong journey of self-discovery** developing and understanding physical/psychological and spiritual needs. It is a discovery of who we are attracted to at various levels and learning from experiences to appropriate strategies towards fulfilment

Positive sexuality

It is useful to consider how you can redress the balance of the missing or negative messages people with learning disabilities receive about their sexuality.

Sexuality reflection sheet

Take some time to reflect on what sexuality means to **you** professionally.

Note down (write or draw):

1 How would **you** define sexuality?

2 What are the factors that **you** think contribute to, or influence the development of, sexuality?

3 What do **you** think the people with learning disabilities that you work with and care for need in order to support the development of their own positive sexuality?

What does sexuality work include?

Using the following model can provide a way for those involved in sexuality work with people with learning disabilities to reflect on the key areas they need to explore for their professional development and the people they work with.

This model also highlights the importance of the specific knowledge, awareness and skills that staff need to work more proactively with people with learning disabilities in sexuality work.

Sexuality work
The key elements

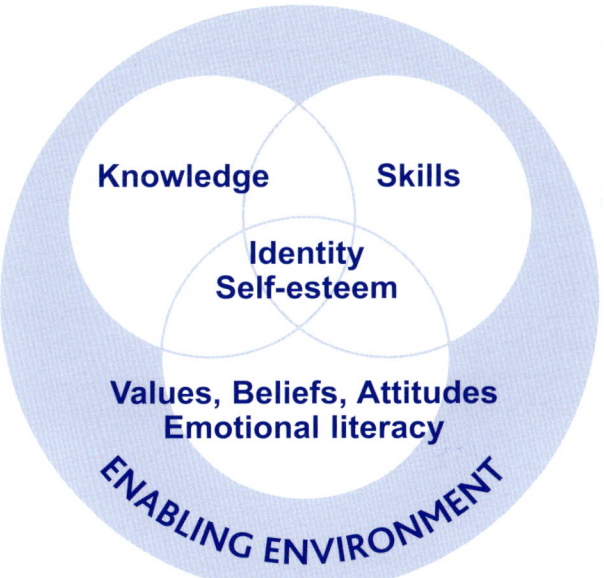

Checklist for sexuality work

A programme of work for people with learning disabilities could include the following areas (in the table overleaf).

Look at each topic area and consider:

- how **relevant (R)** it is for your work
- how **competent (C)** you feel in each area
- how far you **include (I)** it currently in your work.

Use a scale of 1–5, where **1 = low** and **5 = high**.

Knowledge could include:	R	C	I
• puberty – physical changes			
• lifecycle			
• rights and responsibilities			
• confidentiality			
• the law			
• parts of the body – functions			
• sexual activity including masturbation			
• contraception, sexually transmitted infections			
• safer sex			
• pregnancy			
• consent, decision making and rights			
• exploitation.			
Skills could include:			
• assertiveness – saying "yes" and "no"			
• finding a voice and making decisions			
• talking/communicating about sex and relationships			
• relationships – appropriate behaviours in different relationships			
• appropriate public and private behaviours			
• understanding and making informed choices for example, around contraception			
• requesting help from trusted people.			

Awareness/clarification of feelings, beliefs and values could include:	R	C	I
• principles and values for example, religion, culture, family or wider society			
• personal boundaries			
• puberty – emotional changes			
• appropriate feelings in different relationships for example, friendships, marriage and partnerships			
• feeling safe			
• sexual health			
• self-esteem and identity			
• feeling listened to and hearing others			
• sensuality			
• physical pleasure			
• influence of pornography			
• views of others and self for example, parents, religion or wider society			
• feelings about wanting a baby and parenthood			
• attraction and different expectations in relationships			
• managing feelings at the beginning, during and/or at the end of a relationship.			

Total your scores. If you score high for relevance but low for either competence or inclusion, this may point to a training need or a need to revisit and further develop your organisation's sexuality and learning disabilities policy.

Resources to support this work

Staff and carers who are carrying out work based on life skills, empowerment and self-esteem are already doing aspects of sexuality work. If this is coupled with clear organisational sexuality and learning disabilities policies and guidelines, as well as appropriate training and knowledge about existing resources, then these factors can help to accelerate this work. Staff and carers can feel equipped and confident to explore issues and feelings with the people they work with or care for in a constructive and appropriate manner.

There is a range of effective teaching resources that can help staff to cover many of the topic areas in the checklist on previous pages.

Laws, rights and responsibilities

National laws and guidance

People with learning disabilities have the same rights and responsibilities in law as any other person. Exclusions may apply to people with severe learning disabilities who are deemed unable to give consent in law. Their rights are not automatically transferred to carers but in consultation with a range of professionals, decisions can be made about what is in the best interests of the person with learning disabilities.

This section provides brief summaries of key legislation and guidance in England and Wales which relate to every individual, plus those that apply more specifically to people with learning disabilities and their sexuality. For more in-depth information and practical guidance see the FPA book *Learning disabilities, sex and the law: a practical guide*.

Laws and guidance which underpin sexual health and sex and relationships work

Equality Act 2010

The Equality Act 2010 broadens the Equality Act 2006 to include a new equality duty that continues to cover race, gender and disability, and has been extended to cover age, sexual orientation, religion/belief, pregnancy and maternity, and gender reassignment.

Among a range of changes it strengthens the law protecting carers and disabled people from discrimination.[5]

Equality Act 2006

The main provisions of the Equality Act include encouraging and supporting the development of a society in which:

- people's ability to achieve their potential is not limited by prejudice or discrimination
- there is respect for and protection of each individual's human rights
- there is respect for the dignity and worth of each individual
- each individual has an equal opportunity to participate in society, and
- there is mutual respect between groups based on understanding and valuing of diversity and on shared respect for equality and human rights
- people are not discriminated against because of their race, gender, disability, religion or belief, age or sexual orientation.[6]

Mental Capacity Act 2005

The Mental Capacity Act 2005 provides a statutory framework to empower and protect vulnerable people who are not able to make their own decisions. It makes it clear

---

5 Government Equalities Office, *Equality Act 2010: What Do I Need to Know? A Summary Guide for Public Sector Organisations* (Government Equalities Office, 2010).
6 The Commission for Equality and Human Rights, *Equality Act 2006* (The Commission for Equality and Human Rights, 2006).

who can take decisions, in which situations, and how they should go about this.

The Act is underpinned by a set of five key principles:

1 A presumption of capacity – every adult has the right to make his or her own decisions and must be assumed to have the capacity to do so unless it is proved otherwise.

2 The right for individuals to be supported to make their own decisions – people must be given all appropriate help before anyone concludes that they cannot make their own decisions.

3 That individuals must retain the right to make what might be seen as eccentric or unwise decisions.

4 Best interests – anything done for, or on behalf of people without capacity must be in their best interests.

5 Least restrictive intervention – anything done for, or on behalf of people without capacity should be the least restrictive of their basic rights and freedoms.

It is important to note that no decision regarding sexual activity can be made on behalf of someone else.

Consent

A person is considered to have the mental capacity to make choices for themself, thereby giving consent, if they can:

- understand information given to them
- retain that information long enough to be able to make the decision
- weigh up the information available to make the decision
- communicate their decision.[7]

---

7 Great Britain Parliament, Mental Capacity Act 2005 (TSO, 2005).

Valuing people now 2009

Valuing people now: a new three-year strategy for people with learning disabilities was introduced as guidance in 2009 with the aim of improving services for people with learning disabilities across health, housing, employment and community care services.

Valuing people now contains two key messages directly relevant to sexuality and learning disability:

1 **Human rights**
   "People with learning disabilities have the same human rights as everyone else and … adults with learning disabilities are particularly vulnerable to breaches of their human rights."

2 **Relationships and having a family**
   "The importance of enabling people with learning disabilities to meet new people, form all kinds of relationships, and to lead a fulfilling life with access to a diverse range of social and leisure activities … their right to become parents and the need for adequate support to sustain the family unit. There is evidence that people with learning disabilities have limited opportunities to build and maintain social networks and friendships. Parents with a learning disability do not get sufficient access to support, putting families at risk of enforced separation. However, Sure Start children's centres work together with other professionals to help parents with learning disabilities and their children receive the right emotional and practical support to meet the assessed needs of the child and family."[8]

---

8 Department of Health, *Valuing People Now – a Three Year Strategy for People with Learning Disabilities* (Department of Health, 2009).

Laws and guidance which concern sexual health and sex and relationships work

Special Educational Needs and Disability Act 2001 (SENDA)

SENDA established legal rights for disabled students in pre- and post-16 education. It introduced the right for disabled students not to be discriminated against in education, training and any services provided wholly or mainly for students, and for those enrolled on courses provided by 'responsible bodies'.

Forced Marriage (Civil Protection) Act 2007

This Act makes provision for protecting individuals against being forced to enter into marriage without their free and full consent and for protecting individuals who have been forced to enter into marriage without such consent. 'Force' includes being coerced by threats or other psychological means.

Gender Recognition Act 2004

This Act provides transsexual people with legal recognition in their acquired gender. Legal recognition follows from the issue of a full gender recognition certificate by a gender recognition panel. In practical terms, legal recognition has the effect that, for example, a male-to-female transsexual person is legally recognised as a woman in English law. On the issue of a full gender recognition certificate, the person is entitled to a new birth certificate reflecting the acquired gender and is able to marry someone of the opposite gender to his or her acquired gender.

Civil Partnership Act 2004

This Act creates a legal relationship of civil partnership, which two people of the same-sex can form by signing a registration document. It also ensures that same-sex couples who form a civil partnership receive the same treatment in a wide range of legal matters as opposite-sex couples who enter into a civil marriage.

Local Government Act 2003

This Act repealed the homophobic legislation that discriminated against same-sex relationships known as Section 28 of the Local Government Act 1988.

Sexual Offences Act 2003

The Sexual Offences Act 2003 made every offence, except rape, gender neutral, removed homophobic aspects of sexual offences legislation and provided more protection for vulnerable 16 and 17 year olds against exploitation and abuse. It redefined family relationships concerning sex with a child family member aged under 18. Following the equalisation of the age of consent to homosexual acts in the Sexual Offences Amendment Act 2000, it was the first piece of legislation to state that the age of consent is now 16 for any gender and sexual orientation. It also detailed specific legislation to protect people of any age with limited mental capacity from exploitation and abuse. There is guidance to support the Act concerning under age sex and the implications for a range of professionals.

The Sexual Offences Act 2003 refers to 'people with a mental disorder'. Mental disorder is defined by the Mental Health Act 2007 as any disorder or disability of mind, whether permanent or temporary.

The Fraser Guidelines

Gillick v West Norfolk and Wisbech Area Health Authority [1986] AC 112

In England, in 1982, Victoria Gillick sought a High Court ruling against her local area health authority and the Department of Health and Social Security (DHSS) to prevent advice being given to her daughters without her consent. The case was dismissed, but the Appeal Court overturned this in 1984, judging parental consent to be important. An appeal to the House of Lords resulted in DHSS guidance being re-instated in 1985 and the production of guidelines, commonly known as the Fraser Guidelines, which apply in England and Wales.

The Fraser Guidelines are:

> A doctor or other professional can provide sexual health treatment or advice without the parents' knowledge or consent if it is established that:

- the young person understands the advice
- he/she can't be persuaded to inform a parent
- he/she is likely to have sex anyway whether or not the treatment or advice is given
- his/her physical or mental health would suffer without the advice or treatment
- his/her best interests require it.

These guidelines, now embedded into best practice guidance from the Department of Health, exist for all young people including those with learning disabilities who have the capacity to consent to sexual activity.[9]

---

9 Department of Health, *Best Practice Guidance for Doctors and Other Health Professionals on the Provision of Advice and Treatment to Young People Under 16 on Contraception, Sexual and Reproductive Health* (Department of Health, 2004).

Policy development

Consultation with people with learning disabilities, other staff and parents and carers is at the heart of effective policy development. It enables all parties to own and endorse the work if they trust the process. It helps everyone agree their rights and responsibilities. During policy development everyone has a responsibility to respect the rights of others to freedom and choice. It is the duty of staff to promote the rights surrounding informed choice and explain the responsibilities that accompany those choices for people with learning disabilities. It follows that staff need to monitor this process of decision making to ensure that no one involved becomes open to threat, deception or abuse.

Accessible policies for people with learning disabilities

Policies have a major impact on the opportunities and experiences of people with learning disabilities. They should be adapted and written in an accessible way that can be understood and used by people with learning disabilities.

Local policy and guidelines on rights and responsibilities

Local and organisational policy and guidelines on sexuality work and the sexual rights of people with learning disabilities must reflect national legislation, guidance and strategy. They also need to follow the principles of freedom to choose, balanced with protection from harm. This may mean that aspects of privacy, for some people with learning disabilities, may need to be surrendered if their rights to relationships and sexual activity are to be upheld. Every organisation should have a policy and guidelines for staff working with young people and/or adults with learning disabilities regarding personal and social relationships before any form of sexuality work is introduced. This can support the rights, responsibilities and safeguards for all concerned with providing and receiving a service.

From a legal perspective, people who broadly lack the capacity to consent will differ in their rights and responsibilities. However, the following list is useful for staff, carers and people with learning disabilities to consider (using appropriate methods of communication) and work out what acceptable and legal behaviours might look like for each individual.

The rights of adults with learning disabilities can include:

- access to guidance which will assist them in their social, personal and sexual development
- access to support and advice from people who are competent to provide it
- the opportunity to develop close, intimate and loving relationships and the privacy which this demands
- to have appropriate support and protection from exploitation, abuse and degrading treatment
- to have information about himself/herself kept confidential.

The responsibilities of adults with learning disabilities can include:

- to stay within the law as any other citizen
- to respect the rights of others

- to treat others with respect, consideration and sensitivity.

The rights of parents and carers can include:

- to be clear about their role and the support available to them

- to be informed and consulted if the adult with learning disabilities has clearly expressed this as their wish

- to have appropriate support and protection from exploitation, abuse and degrading treatment that may be perpetrated by the people they care for

- to be treated with respect, consideration and sensitivity

- not to be held responsible for the action of the adult with learning disabilities.

The responsibilities of parents can include:

- to work constructively with others involved in supporting the adult with learning disabilities as agreed in the care plan or any other agreement

- to treat their relative with respect and consideration

- to make a distinction between what is in the best interest of their relative with learning disabilities and what is in their own best interest

- to support and promote positive sexual health and relationships for the person with learning disabilities and to respect their relationship choices and preferences

- to keep the services supporting them informed where appropriate.

The rights of staff and managers can include:

- to have appropriate support and protection from exploitation, abuse and degrading treatment which may be perpetrated by the person with learning disabilities

- to be given relevant information, advice, support, supervision, and training from someone who is appropriately skilled and conversant with policy on personal and social relationships

- to be treated with respect, consideration and sensitivity

- to be protected from unfair allegations and adverse publicity, and to be supported when allegations are made, by means of policies and procedures.

The responsibilities of staff and managers can include:

- to work constructively with others within policies and procedures to support adults with learning disabilities in pursuing personal and social relationships

- to report any incidents of abuse, neglect or poor practice in line with their employers' adult protection procedures in a non-judgemental manner

- to request training, support and guidance where necessary

- to ensure that the adult with learning disabilities is kept informed and treated with respect and dignity and appropriate confidentiality in a non-abusive, non-judgemental environment.

Individual rights of people with learning disabilities

The following list does not advocate a universal application of every right if it puts individuals at risk. The rights of people with a learning disability need to be viewed as part of the range of rights every citizen should be eligible for. These can include:

The right to be supported in making informed choices and give consent about relationships and sexual activity under the Mental Capacity Act 2005
Staff need to ensure that they have a clear strategy for every individual they work with to assess capacity for each situation where informed choices and decisions need to be made.

The right to find out about what is meant by sexuality, and opportunities to build the skills and awareness needed to develop this core aspect of identity in positive ways
This requires staff and carers to be competent in delivering this wide area of work. Those working with people with learning disabilities have a duty to assess what information each individual in their care is ready to assimilate and what skills and awareness they are ready to explore. Staff need to recognise their duty of care and the entitlements of those they work with under the law.

The right to engage in mutually consensual sexual activity within the law; and the right to choose not to engage in any sexual activity
The same restrictions that the law places on everyone regarding sexual activity should also apply to people with learning disabilities. Sexual activity should not occur in places that may offend people or be abusive. Nor should there be an expectation that people with learning disabilities *must* engage in sexual activity or have any more right than anyone else to have sexual relationships.

Staff members' duty of care requires that protection from harm and freedom to enjoy rights are balanced by clear monitoring processes about being able to give consent and make informed decisions.

The right to access sexual health advice and services that enable individuals to make informed choices about protecting their sexual health
There is no suggestion that it is right to impose contraception – sterilisation is contraception – onto someone because others believe that it is necessary to do so. This would be unlawful. However, protection from pregnancy and/or infection can be dealt with via preventative educational work and support to access appropriate sexual health services.

The right to get married, form a civil partnership or form an ongoing sexual relationship
This applies where an informed decision is made and consent is clearly given by all involved parties. If there is any suspicion of threat or deception it must be investigated. Staff need to be aware of the legal aspects of marriage and the Civil Partnership Act 2006.

The right for pregnant women to choose to keep the baby, have the baby adopted or have an abortion
Staff have a responsibility to provide information and advice on sex and relationships that can enable people with learning disabilities to make informed choices about their reproductive rights. This means that, where appropriate, individuals should be supported to discuss and express their understanding of reproductive rights and responsibilities. Also, where appropriate, people should be helped to develop necessary parenting skills. In situations where babies may be taken into care or there are potential genetic issues, counselling and education should be provided. The right to choose adoption and abortion should also be supported.

The right not to be sexually abused, threatened or exploited and to be protected from sexual abuse

In a society where people with learning disabilities are so commonly devalued, it is important to reiterate this basic right and make explicit the behaviour that could constitute even mild abuse. Protection can also mean that people with learning disabilities are empowered through education to seek help and say "no" if coerced into activities they do not like. Rights to protection are clearly defined in the Sexual Offences Act 2003 and should directly inform practice/service delivery.

Sexuality policy checklist

The checklist below gives a basic list of areas that could be addressed to support positive sexualities while providing safeguards for all involved. During a policy development training session use the checklist to map what your policy currently covers and what needs to be developed.

What is in your policy?	Yes	No	Needs to be developed
1 Introduction			
• Who you are and what you do (your service).			
2 Evidence base as to what sexuality work is and why it is important			
• Rationale – what is it, what are the benefits, what is the evidence?			

What is in your policy?
(continued)

	Yes	No	Needs to be developed
• How it relates to other work for example, life skills and emotional health.			
• Aims.			
3 Law, policy, guidance and duties			
• Strategic partnerships.			
• Local partnership boards.			
• Rights and entitlements.			
• Responsibilities.			
• Duty of care.			
• Mental capacity.			
• Consent.			
• Protection of vulnerable adults.			
4 Guidance on specific issues			
• Public and private behaviours.			
• Inappropriate sexualised behaviour.			
• Masturbation.			
• Intimate touching – safe and unsafe.			
• Sexual relationships.			

What is in your policy?
(continued)

	Yes	No	Needs to be developed
• Sharing a room with a partner.			
• Gender issues.			
• Transgender identities.			
• Transvestism.			
• Sexual orientation – heterosexual, homosexual, bisexual.			
• Marriage, civil partnership, co-habitation.			
• Pregnancy choices including keeping the baby, having the baby adopted and abortion.			
• Parenthood.			
• Contraception, including male and female sterilisation.			
• Safer sex and condom use.			
• Sexually transmitted infections.			
• Ethnicity, culture and religion.			
• Pornography.			
• Any other issues.			

What is in your policy? *(continued)*	Yes	No	Needs to be developed
5 Supporting and protecting staff			
• Inappropriate behaviour from people with learning disabilities, and others.			
• Reporting sexual abuse.			
• Supervision.			
• Sexuality 'expert' within the team.			
• Reporting procedures.			
• 'Dilemmas' expert panel.			
• Training.			
• Access to resources.			
6 Partnership work			
• Parents.			
• Other agencies.			
• Other services.			
7 Monitoring and evaluation			
• Who will monitor the implementation of the policy?			
• How will the work be evaluated?			
• When will it be next reviewed (once every two to three years is advisable)?			

Local guidelines and policy on anti-discriminatory practice

Guided by law, policy, strategy and duties, staff should be working in an anti-discriminatory way in all areas of work and for all people with learning disabilities. People may face multiple areas of discrimination if they are from a particular black or minority ethnic or cultural community, religious background or class, or if they identify themselves as lesbian, gay, bisexual or transgender.

When working in the area of sexuality, staff need to understand the person with learning disabilities' social, ethnic and cultural background and whether or not they wish to retain or change these influences. It is part of a staff member's professional role to provide diverse experiences for all people with learning disabilities. Creating opportunities to explore identities within an inclusive framework is central to this work.

It is also important for staff to challenge discrimination, whenever appropriate, in local communities and to promote positive images of people with learning disabilities within this wider context.

> "I have learnt how to evaluate my own beliefs and values and how to put these aside and work in an open-minded manner."
>
> **FPA Learning Disabilities Roadshow participant**

Working agreement/ground rules

Forming a working agreement is the cornerstone of developing anti-discriminatory practice when working with individuals or groups of people with learning disabilities, other staff members or carers. These help make explicit how people should treat each other and expect to be treated.

The individual or group can therefore feel valued and heard within an inclusive environment.

Working agreement/ground rules for running groups or doing individual educational work with people with learning disabilities

Below is an example of a working agreement developed and agreed with a group of people with learning disabilities:

- Information about you belongs to you. It is your choice who you tell.

- Information about other people belongs to them. It is their choice who they tell.

- We will try to use language we can all understand so choose your own words.

- If you don't understand anything, ask.

- It is helpful if you are able to say, able to show, sign, draw …

    "I think …"

    "I feel …"

    "I want …"

    "I like …"

    "I don't like …"

- What you say to us is private unless you or someone else might not be safe. I will tell you first if I think I need to talk to someone else, I will be honest with you.

- We might not always agree – people think different things and that is okay.

- We will try to make a safe space.

Checklist for a working agreement
Having reflected on the working agreement above, which points might be useful to use with the groups of people or individuals with learning disabilities you work with?

How might you put together a working agreement with the people you work with?

List any key points you might like to discuss and talk them through with the people that you work with.

Boundaries

If you discuss issues that are likely to come up, before they come up, it is possible to clarify boundaries and form clear guidelines that can support and protect both people with learning disabilities and staff, when carrying out sexuality work.

The following statements could be explored as part of a workplace training session. Look at potential positive and negative aspects to these statements. In adding your own additional context you will be able to create a much wider picture of what is or is not acceptable for the people you work with.

Boundaries and guidelines development statements

Please note: The following nine statements are deliberately provocative – they are not recommendations of what should be put into practice.

Statement 1:
Allowing mild unwanted sexual advances between people with learning disabilities enables the recipient to learn assertiveness skills.

Statement 2:
It is useful to discourage intimate relationships between people with learning disabilities when it is evident to staff that there is no long-term future for the couple.

Statement 3:
Pornography is an acceptable form of personal SRE for people with learning disabilities.

Statement 4:
If people with learning disabilities are influenced by limiting parental values and beliefs about sexuality, it becomes the responsibility of staff to provide more diverse perspectives.

Statement 5:
Demonstrations of affection between people with learning disabilities of the same sex are less acceptable in public than between people of the opposite sex.

Statement 6:
All people with learning disabilities, regardless of sexual orientation, require information about marriage, pregnancy and parenthood.

Statement 7:
Staff should always encourage people with learning disabilities to explore their sexual needs and feelings.

Statement 8:
All people with learning disabilities need to be informed of the variety of behaviours that constitute sexual abuse.

Statement 9:
Masturbation in a public part of the house can be tolerated if no other service user is there, or likely to be present.

This exercise is used regularly on FPA training courses and participants' opinions vary greatly.

STATEMENT 1:
Allowing mild unwanted sexual advances between people with learning disabilities enables the recipient to learn assertiveness skills.

The spectrum of opinion included:

- This is completely unacceptable. Any form of sexual advance that is unwanted should be dealt with by staff.

- Empowerment requires skills to be practised. If a service user was taught assertiveness skills and expressed a desire to deal with the unwanted advances it would require staff support. Risk-taking in a controlled environment may be preferable to 'throwing people in at the deep end' unsupervised.

STATEMENT 2:
It is useful to discourage intimate relationships between people with learning disabilities when it is evident to staff that there is no long-term future for the couple.

Opinion focused on:

- All service users have the same right to be in a relationship with few long-term possibilities as anyone else. Safeguards would come in the form of staff checking out that there is no exploitation or abuse in the situation.

STATEMENT 3:
Pornography is an acceptable form of personal SRE for people with learning disabilities.

The spectrum of opinion included:

- Pornography can show women and men in submissive and objectified roles and can give a negative message.

- Pornography is a choice that can be respected with safeguards, namely that staff do not provide pornography but support its use by explaining that it can only be used in a private space, for example a person with learning disabilities could have satellite television in their bedroom and this could be monitored by staff in terms of agreed times for watching pornography. They should also be encouraged to participate in other activities during the day.

- Proactive discussions about women and getting consent for sex would need to occur as part of sexuality work.

STATEMENT 4:
If people with learning disabilities are influenced by limiting parental values and beliefs about sexuality, it becomes the responsibility of staff to provide more diverse perspectives.

The spectrum of opinion included:

- We need to work with parents to explain the benefits of SRE and the rights of people with learning disabilities. As people with learning disabilities often visit or live with their parents, any new skills, awareness or information that staff provide needs to take into account who people live with or visit regularly.

- Providing diverse perspectives is useful only if it is tailored to the individual. So, if exactly the same information is given to all people with learning disabilities it could equally prove destructive if it is not appropriate to their needs.

STATEMENT 5:
Demonstrations of affection between people with learning disabilities of the same sex are less acceptable in public than between people of the opposite sex.

The spectrum of opinion included:

- The rights of people of every sexual orientation to express affection must be supported.

- The law and society still discriminate against people who are gay showing affection in public, so teaching people with learning disabilities this fact and the reality of discrimination is necessary for their protection.

STATEMENT 6:
All people with learning disabilities, regardless of sexual orientation, require information about marriage, pregnancy and parenthood.

The spectrum of opinion included:

- All people with learning disabilities need this information even if they never experience any of these situations first hand.

STATEMENT 7:
Staff should always encourage people with learning disabilities to explore their sexual needs and feelings.

The spectrum of opinion included:

- Some people with learning disabilities might just want a special friend without wanting to become sexually intimate with them.

- While exploring sexual needs and feelings could be encouraged it should not always have to happen, only when appropriate.

- It is vital for some people with learning disabilities as their aggressive behaviour has been shown to decline when educated about dealing with sexual frustration.

STATEMENT 8:
All people with learning disabilities need to be informed of the variety of behaviours that constitute sexual abuse.

The spectrum of opinion included:

- Talking about it to all people with learning disabilities might scare some of them.

- You must be prepared with an agreed process or plan if someone discloses that they are being or have been abused.

- There needs to be a programme developed to inform people with learning disabilities what are appropriate behaviours from a range of people involved in their lives.

- This must be coupled with assertiveness work, for example expressing (verbally or otherwise) "no" to unwanted touches or anything they are not sure of and stating what they want until they are able to talk to a trusted person.

STATEMENT 9:
Masturbation in a public part of the house can be tolerated if no other service user is there, or likely to be present.

The spectrum of opinion included:

- This must be discouraged as it gives a mixed message about public places.

- Masturbation in private should be discussed and enabled where necessary.

Spheres of influence 5

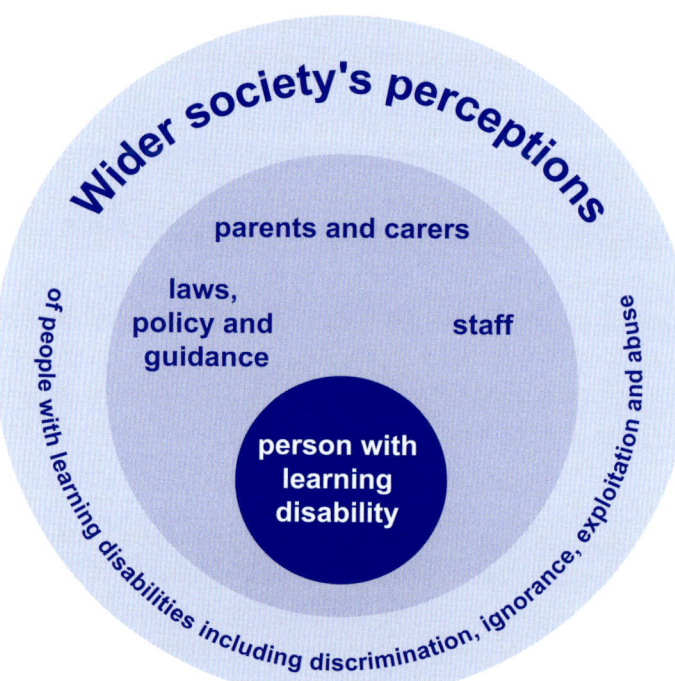

Where can professionals bring about change?

The diagram above is a useful way of looking at what influences the lives of people with learning disabilities. It shows three spheres. The outer sphere represents wider society's perceptions. The inner sphere represents influences from parents, carers, staff and the law. At the core is the person with learning disabilities.

Unlike their non-disabled peers many people with learning disabilities will not have access to extensive social opportunities. Most of their learning will have come from a smaller network of people, including parents, carers and staff from a wide variety of services.

Messages about friendships, relationships and sexuality may be omitted or filtered, through a sincere desire to protect individuals from exploitation and abuse. This may limit their knowledge within the inner sphere of influence and have an impact on the person with learning disabilities' choices.

The outer sphere of influence represents society's exclusion of any disability. Staff do not have control over this outer sphere which represents discrimination faced by those with a learning disability. Therefore, staff should focus their attention on working within the inner sphere to develop consistent skills and awareness with people with learning disabilities. This will aim to uphold rights and fulfil their duty of care.

Working with individuals or groups to build a map of key people, institutions and rules that influence their lives can focus attention on creating a fully enabling environment to work in. It also serves to create a manageable challenge for staff. This in turn can lead to using national policy to influence more effective service delivery. It is also helpful to use national legislation that bans for example, hate crimes and sexual exploitation against people with learning disabilities. This can help to confront and deal with negative perceptions and discrimination of people with learning disabilities within society.

Working with parents

Working in partnership with the parents of people with learning disabilities is an essential staff role. It is important to recognise that parents' behaviours which are seen as restrictive will usually be driven by the very positive intention of protection. If staff acknowledge that fear and grief could lie behind a parent's protective impulse it may lead to better dialogue with parents who are opposed to sexuality work.

> "Bringing up a child, who is not 'perfect' in the eyes of the world, often instigates a period of grieving for the 'lost child' that is, the child you were expecting but did not have. How the diagnosis is given and the disability explained is crucial to how well parents are able to deal with this situation emotionally and intellectually.
>
> Families who are unable to grieve can become stuck and this can block the idea that their child could ever reach any form of maturity. Expressions of grief may be felt throughout the whole of the child's life not just immediately after diagnosis.
>
> Having the opportunity to express the sadness and the grief over not having the child expected can help parents to move forward. The more parents are able to come to terms with the disability of their son or daughter the more they may then be able to accept them as sexual beings." [10]

---

10 Drury J, Hutchinson L and Wright J, *Holding On, Letting Go* (Souvenir Press, 2000).

Working with the concerns of parents and carers about doing sexuality work

> "I realised that I have personal feelings but to fulfil my role responsibly I must listen to all perspectives, from the person with learning disabilities to their parents and other colleagues, and be broadminded and empathetic."
>
> **FPA Learning Disabilities Roadshow participant**

Staff need a range of knowledge, skills and awareness to liaise and negotiate with parents who may have doubts about the value of sexuality work. Parents or carers may approach staff with fear, anxiety and mistrust based on past experiences where the person they care for may have been left open to exploitation or abuse.

There may have been situations where staff ignored parents' concerns because they did not feel equipped to deal with issues such as masturbation.

Skills and awareness checklist

This checklist can be used for continuing professional development to help you reflect on the skills you may find useful when taking on board parents'/carers' feelings about sexuality work.

Where you have ticked 'Yes', use the third column to give some examples. Where you have ticked 'No', use the third column to consider what you might need to do.

Skills and awareness	Yes	No	Examples or ideas
1 The emotional Do I … ?			
• Listen to emotional and sometimes irrational statements and still allow the parent or carer to feel heard and understood?			
• Demonstrate empathy by showing that I am able to put myself in their situation and view the issue as they do?			
• Demonstrate active listening by using open questions to widen the conversation?			
• Reflect back what parents have said to allow them to confirm that I have heard and understood their views?			
• Ensure I am honest by being realistic, that is, not being tempted to reassure if there is nothing concrete to back this up or if it will infringe the person with learning disabilities' rights?			
• Maintain clear communication with my organisation to ensure that I feel supported (by manager, colleagues, policy) to give information, realistic advice and reassurance?			

| Skills and awareness
(continued)	Yes	No	Examples or ideas
2 The rational Do I know … ?			
● About information relevant to the situation?			
● Relevant aspects of a wide range of legislation?			
● About national strategy for example, *Valuing people now 2009*?			
● About local policies, guidance and procedures on equality and sexuality?			
● And understand my professional boundaries?			
● And understand my duty of care around entitlements to sexuality work for people with learning disabilities?			
● Rights and responsibilities of colleagues, parents and people with learning disabilities?			
3 Personal skills Am I able to … ?			
● Show that I value the parent or carer while being honest about their opinions – if they are discriminatory?			

Skills and awareness *(continued)*	Yes	No	Examples or ideas
3 Personal skills *(continued)* Am I able to … ?			
• Demonstrate understanding?			
• Maintain my professional cool in the face of potential conflict?			
• Resist acting on assumptions so that I can check out what the parent means, as misunderstandings can be destructive?			
• Maintain clarity in explaining the rationale for sexuality work in order to build trust?			
• Mediate and facilitate around difficult behaviours?			

Working with reluctant colleagues

Staff need clear guidance about professional boundaries in order to carry out sexuality work with people with learning disabilities.

Without policy or training it is possible that some staff may allow their personal beliefs to influence how they carry out sexuality work. This is a potentially discriminatory situation that may ignore and deny a duty of care. In tackling staff reluctance it is important to listen to their concerns and allow time to provide explanations about the nature of this work.

As with any emotive situation, it is important that staff fear and anxiety is heard and responded to appropriately before the benefits of sexuality work can be put forward.

The following statements could be explored as part of a workplace training session. Look at and discuss potential positive and negative aspects of these statements. In adding your own additional context you will be able to create a much wider picture of what is or is not acceptable for the people you work with.

Reluctant colleagues statements

Potential barriers posed by reluctant staff and ways of responding

Here are some statements made by colleagues who could be seen as reluctant to engage in sexuality work.

Read each one and imagine you are the person whose role it is to deal with other colleagues' concerns about sexuality work – then consider the following for each statement.

- How do you **feel** about someone making this statement?

  This is your personal gut-reaction.

- What do you **think** about the statement?

  This is your professional reflection on the potential emotions and the rational explanation you need to give them.

- What would you **do** in reply to this statement?

  This is your measured professional response that recognises the need to engage with both the emotional and rational aspects of your colleague's statement.

1. Doing this work will put ideas into their heads, they only have the mental age of children so it would encourage them to have sex.

2. It is against my religion to condone sex out of marriage, I would feel compromised.

3. The parents would not allow it.

4. It's all very well to talk about their rights but we don't know the first thing about this work.

5. Some of them have been abused; we don't want to open a 'can of worms'.

6. Some of them try to harass and abuse the others, talking about sex will just make it worse.

7. Are you saying we should encourage them to have sex, what if someone gets pregnant? I don't want to have to tell the parents.

8. I don't want to get into talking about gay and lesbian stuff.

9. I don't want to teach someone to masturbate.

10. Why do I have to do it?

11. Who or what will support me? Will I get training?

After you have completed this exercise look at some of the responses overleaf that could be made when discussing this work with reluctant colleagues.

1. **Doing this work will put ideas into their heads, they only have the mental age of children so it would encourage them to have sex.**

    - **Emotional:** I can see you feel very strongly about this ... tell me about your concerns.

    - **Rational:** Mental age does not necessarily have a bearing on someone's capacity to consent. People with learning disabilities should be enabled to enjoy their rights as individuals under the law. They should be helped to make informed choices coupled with their right to protection and freedom from discrimination.

2. **It is against my religion to condone sex out of marriage, I would feel compromised.**

    - **Emotional:** Tell me about your religion.

    - **Rational:** Religions have set codes of conduct and they also usually have a pastoral brief to support individuals even if they have contravened the rules. In any work situation your personal attitudes cannot take precedence over your professional duty of care, which may not conform to your personal beliefs. This kind of behaviour could be construed as discriminatory against the person with learning disabilities.

3. **The parents would not allow it.**

    - **Emotional:** What has been your experience of working with these parents? How do you feel about their behaviour?

- **Rational:** Whose rights must we primarily uphold under the law? Our duty of care is to the person with learning disabilities but it would also include dialogue with parents who hold a significant position of influence. We may, as a staff group, need to explore how we deal with the fear and grief that parents may experience that hampers the development of this work.

4 **It's all very well to talk about their rights but we don't know the first thing about this work.**

- **Emotional:** What do you think this work involves? What might you feel particularly uncomfortable talking about?

- **Rational:** Sexuality work involves for example, life skills – you are already doing this and it is transferable. We will make sure you will have a policy and guidance that you can discuss and also that there is good quality training available. (Note: give honest reassurance and never bring reluctant colleagues into this work without a guarantee of policy, guidance and training.)

5 **Some of them have been abused; we don't want to open a 'can of worms'.**

- **Emotional:** Tell me about the types of general behaviour people who have been abused display. How do you feel about dealing with that?

- **Rational:** We will need to plan one-to-one work and general sexuality work that is distanced and practical for example, exploring acceptable public and private behaviours, making decisions such as saying "no" to unwanted attention, what consent means and how to seek advice.

6 **Some of them try to harass and abuse the others, talking about sex will just make it worse.**

- **Emotional:** I understand and share your fears. If we do not tackle this appropriately it could prove more difficult.

- **Rational:** Again we need to plan one-to-one work and general sexuality work that is distanced and practical for example, exploring acceptable public and private behaviours, making decisions such as saying "no" to unwanted attention, what consent means and how to seek help and advice.

7 **Are you saying we should encourage them to have sex, what if someone gets pregnant? I don't want to have to tell the parents.**

- **Emotional:** I understand your reluctance to do this. Tell me what you think this work is about.

- **Rational:** Let me reassure you that doing this work is not about encouragement but meeting people's needs appropriately. We need to be prepared to give information about pregnancy, contraception and planning families. We also need to look at ideas for engaging parents in sexuality work and provide reassurance about the roles and responsibilities of the staff member.

8 **I don't want to get into talking about gay and lesbian stuff.**

- **Emotional:** What are your concerns in discussing these issues?

- **Rational:** People have choices and offering the right amount of information about homosexuality at the right time can be empowering. In any work situation your personal attitudes cannot take precedence over your professional duty of care, which may not conform to your personal beliefs. This kind of behaviour could be construed as discriminatory against the person with learning disabilities. It is illegal to discriminate on the grounds of sexual orientation.

9 **I don't want to teach someone to masturbate.**

- **Emotional:** What would most concern you if you were asked to do this?

- **Rational:** Not everyone would be expected to do this. There are many ways of teaching this that do not involve physical contact such as using line drawings or videos and talking it through. At the very least we would want all staff to support those who are teaching about masturbation by being positive if asked a question by a person with learning disabilities, even if you then pass them on to someone else.

10 Why do I have to do it?

- **Emotional:** What concerns you about having to take this on as part of your role?

- **Rational:** As before, it will include our duty of care, anti-discriminatory practice, offering informed choice and appropriately promoting the sexual rights of people with learning disabilities.

11 Who or what will support me? Will I get training?

- **Emotional:** What support and training do you feel you would need? Who and what would you like to support you?

- **Rational:** Sexuality work involves for example, life skills – you are already doing this and it is transferable. We will make sure you will have a policy and guidance that you can discuss and also that there is good quality training available.
(Note: Give honest reassurance about policy, guidance, training, supervision and support. Dealing with the emotional – fears and concerns – takes time and understanding.)

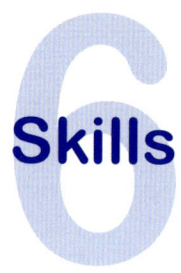

Skills

Communication

Language and service users

The context of words and language is very important. A word used in a particular, possibly derogatory, manner may have a very different emphasis when being used between friends to express something than when used in the workplace.

The use of language can be one of the main areas of concern for staff when working with people with learning disabilities. Tips include:

- establish your levels of language when starting work with a group

- discuss all the words that can be used for different sexual activities and private body parts and come to a common consensus on what is acceptable

- make sure that the words you are using are understood by the group

- make sure you correctly interpret the words the group use

- the more you use a word, the less embarrassing it can become, try some exercises around making the words more everyday for people

- establish that the words which are used in the group may not be appropriate for use in situations outside the group

- make sure your working agreement has a point about appropriate language.

Skills teaching

The process of teaching a new skill to someone with a learning disability takes careful thought, planning and execution.

As a useful staff training exercise look at how to simplify language and instructions to explain a step-by-step process for one of the following:

- male/female condom use

- sanitary towel use

- tampon use.

Consider the information service users need, in addition to the 'how to'. You will need to be creative and could use pictures with verbal explanations, models or visual demonstrations. When delivering the step-by-step processes to people with learning disabilities, they could be carried out over a series of weeks, not just in one session.
Certain points may need repetition and further explanation. Overleaf are examples of step-by-step processes.

Male condom use

1 What is a condom?

- show condoms in and out of packets

- explain that contraception is free for women and men of all ages through the National Health Service. Explain that you can get condoms from contraception and sexual health clinics and young people's services, and some general practices and genitourinary medicine (GUM) clinics (you may need to accompany the service user for the first time). You can buy them from a pharmacy, by mail order or online as well as from vending machines, supermarkets, garages and other shops.

- explain what they do – help prevent pregnancy and help protect against sexually transmitted infections.

2 When should they be used?

- explain when – put the condom on when the penis is fully erect and before it touches the vagina or genital area.

- make this explicit – it is a male form of contraception for use on the erect penis only.

3 Checking your condom

- talk about checking for the date.

4 How to use

- how to open the packet – no rings or sharp things and not with the teeth

- how to ensure it is the right way up – see Top tips

- how to roll a condom onto the erect penis – demonstrate with model, remember to hold the teat at the top of the condom to leave space for sperm

- when it is okay to have sex – when the condom has rolled comfortably to the end of the erect penis.

5 Afterwards

- explain withdrawal – ensure the condom is held securely at the bottom
- explain removal – ensure the sperm is in the condom
- explain disposal – wrapped up in the bin, not down the toilet.

6 What if something goes wrong?

- discuss problems putting condoms on – use another, always make sure you have plenty
- discuss what to do if one splits or comes off – tell someone or go to the contraception clinic or doctor
- only ever use a condom once.

●●●●●●●●● **Top tips** ●●●●●●●●●

One of the most difficult parts of this demonstration is explaining which way up the condom needs to go. Practise in advance – close your eyes and feel around the edges, when it is the right way up you can feel a textured edge and the wrong way is very smooth.

Make sure you have lots of condoms for the group to try with condom demonstrators and also some to take home if they want to practise.

Condom demonstrators are better to use than vegetables (less abstract) – you can buy them as part of the FPA *Contraceptive display kit*.

Female condom use

1 What is a female condom?

- show condoms in and out of packets

- explain that contraception is free for women and men of all ages through the National Health Service. Explain that you can get condoms from contraception and sexual health clinics and young people's services, and some general practices and genitourinary medicine (GUM) clinics (you may need to accompany the service user for the first time). You can buy them from a pharmacy, by mail order or online.

- explain what they do – help prevent pregnancy and help protect against sexually transmitted infections.

2 When should it be used?

- explain when – you can put the condom in any time before sex but always before the penis touches the vagina or genital area.

- make explicit – it is a female form of contraception for use in the vagina only.

3 Where is it used?

- discuss female body parts – external and internal. Describe where the cervix is and how the female condom acts as a barrier.

4 How to use

- how to open the packet – no rings, sharp objects and not with teeth

- what it feels like – very lubricated

- explain why it looks like it does – inner ring sits against the cervix, the outer ring stays outside the vagina
- describe insertion – use a model or visual diagrams
- explain when it is ready to use – note that during sex the man's penis needs to be guided into the female condom to ensure it does not go outside it.

5 Afterwards

- removal – after the man has come, the female condom must be gently removed by twisting the end to keep the sperm in
- explain disposal – wrapped in tissue in the bin, not down the toilet.

"Learning how to handle a female condom without it 'getting away' will never be forgotten!"

FPA Learning Disabilities Roadshow participant

Top tips

The female condom is likely to be a difficult form of contraception for a woman with a learning disability to use.

You may need to work with women on the skills needed to use a female condom and doing some exercises around pinching and twisting might be useful.

Buy vaginal models for this type of work to help make things more visually comprehensive (they are good for tampon work too).

Sanitary towel use (pads, pantyliners)

1 Periods and when to use sanitary towels

- talk about periods, monthly cycles, why sanitary towels are used and the different names for them.

2 What are sanitary towels?

- show different types of sanitary towel, different absorbencies, winged and non-winged
- explain where to get them from (see Top tips).

3 How to use a sanitary towel

- explain processes such as the following:

    1 Go to the toilet – this must be done in private.

    2 Wash hands and go into the cubicle with a sanitary towel.

    3 Take down lower clothes and knickers.

    4 Sit on the toilet and unwrap it (if it has a covering).

    5 Take off the strip of paper covering the sticky back and place the sanitary towel onto the gusset of the knickers with the sticky side down (this may need some practical help to ensure it is stuck in the correct place – see Top tips).

    6 If it has wings, peel off the strips of paper, fold the wings under the gusset and stick down.

    7 Pull knickers and lower clothes up.

    8 Wash hands.

4 Changing and disposal

- explain changing – that sanitary towels will need to be changed depending on the flow of your period and time of day

- explain disposal – sanitary towels need to be disposed of carefully – think about all the different situations clients may be in when changing their sanitary towel and explain that it should be as discreet as possible.

●●●●●●●●● Top tips ●●●●●●●●●

You can make this work special for women by bringing in make up bags and knickers and allowing the group to choose a pair of knickers and some sanitary towels to keep as their own.

The winged sanitary towels tend to be better for service users as they move around less – do some preliminary work on which side is sticky and where it should go – it is good to do this with actual knickers.

Try asking a local supermarket if you could take a group in to show them how the towels are packaged, what they cost, where to find them and what the different types are.

Tampon use

1 Periods and when to use tampons

- talk about periods, monthly cycles and why tampons are used
- explain choice – why they are sometimes used instead of sanitary towels.

2 What are tampons?

- show different types of tampon, applicator and non-applicator, and sizes
- describe where to get tampons from.

3 How to use a tampon

- describe process – see the visual presentation on page 70.

4 Changing and disposal

- explain tampon changing – how often they should be changed
- give women a chart so they can check they have changed their tampons

	Getting up	Lunchtime	Teatime	Bedtime
Day 1				
Day 2				
Day 3				
Day 4				
Day 5				

- explain disposal – in the bin wrapped in tissue, not down the toilet.

"I have much more confidence and experience of demonstration techniques."

FPA Learning Disabilities Roadshow participant

Top tips

Some women with learning disabilities only ever use sanitary towels, not by choice, but because they have never been given another option. Tampons can provide an alternative option in suitable situations.

Be careful if using fake blood (or red water) with tampon demonstrations, some women get very upset by this.

Do bear in mind associated health risks if tampons are not changed regularly, for example, toxic shock syndrome. This will need to be dealt with carefully so as not to scare the women.

Example of simple diagrams to illustrate how to use tampons

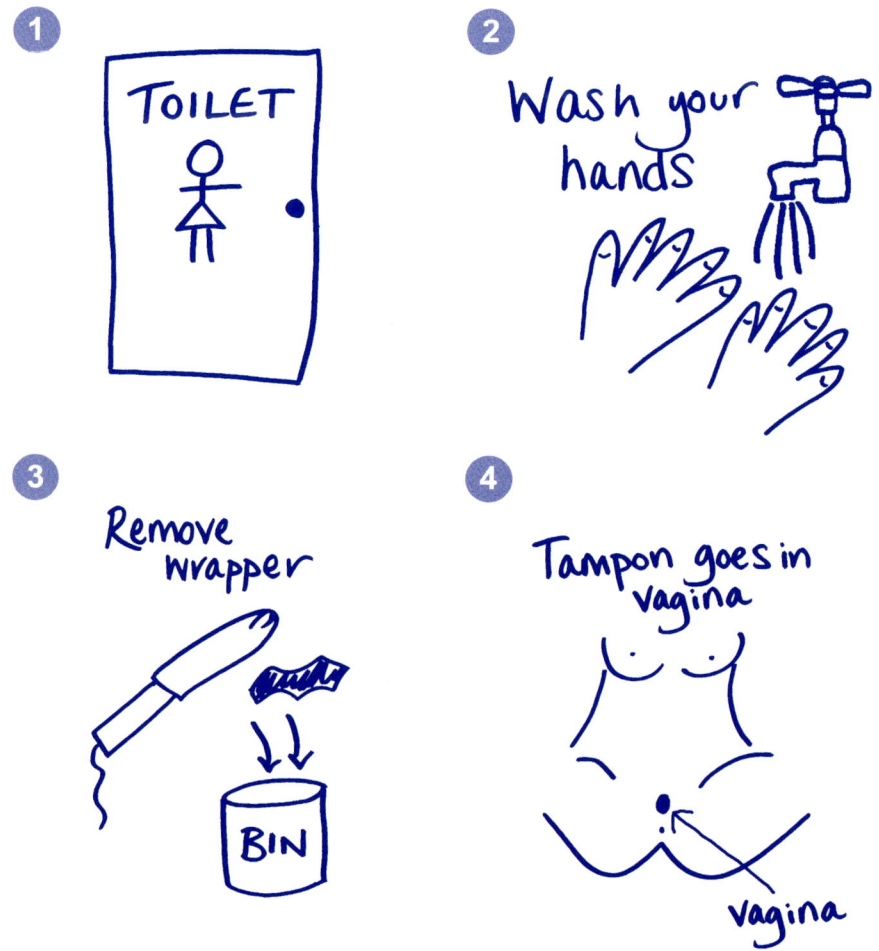

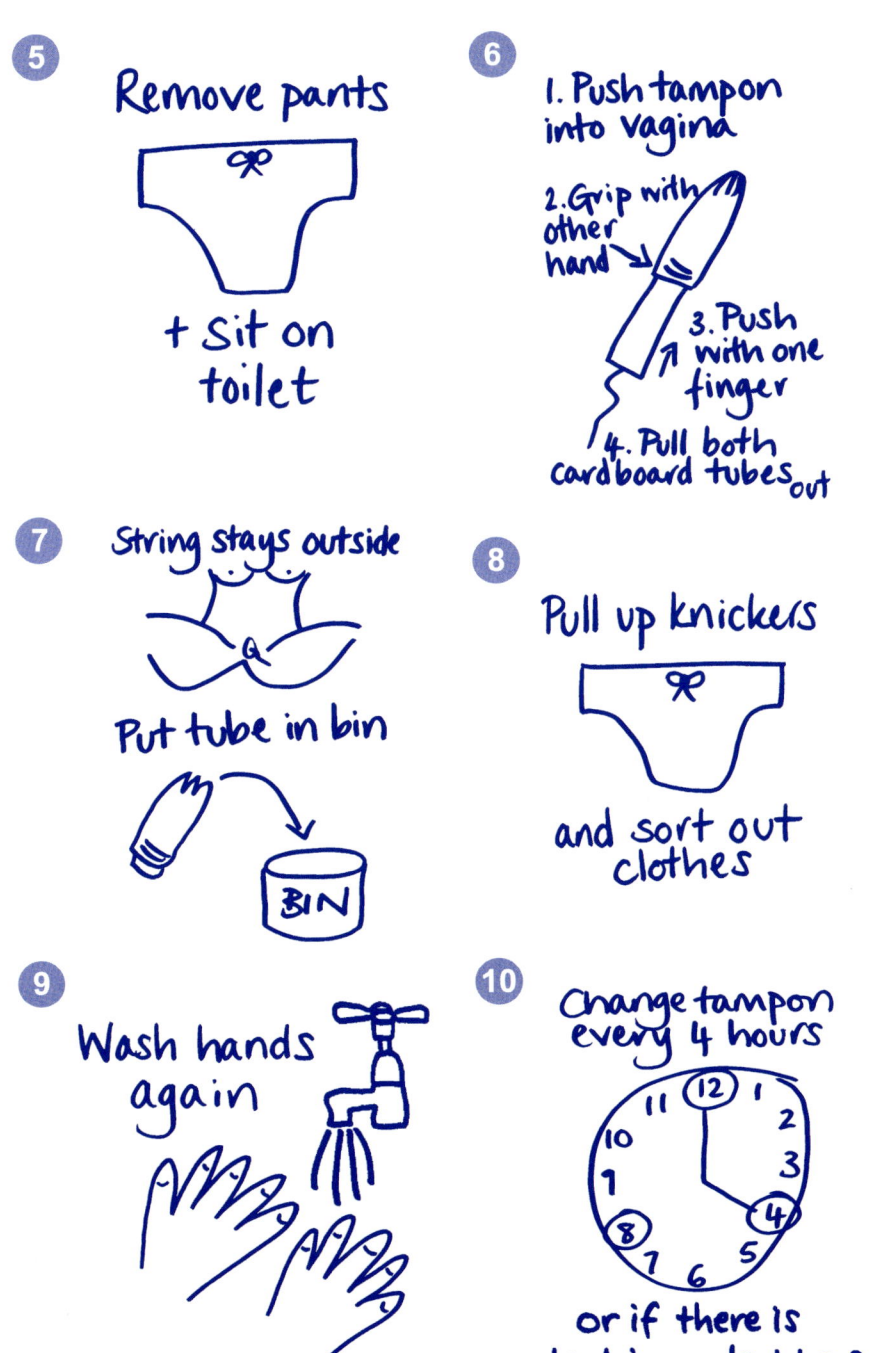

7 Conclusion

Staff and carers who work with people with learning disabilities have to balance the rights of those they work alongside with the need to protect vulnerable individuals from sexual exploitation and abuse. The government has consulted and debated the rights of people with learning disabilities to equitable treatment more fully in the last decade. With changes in legislation and strategies, staff and carers need opportunities to explore national and local guidance. They then need to attend updated training and continue to get support to work effectively and inclusively.

In looking at the law, national policy, rights, responsibilities, dilemmas and practice issues within this guide we anticipate that it will support continuing professional development. Using the checklists and ideas for discussion can provide a series of short sessions to maintain an anti-discriminatory approach to the work that values individual needs. We hope that this guide will also provide a valuable additional resource for staff and carers attending sexuality training.

FPA has been providing sexuality training for staff, carers and parents for decades. This continues to offer a clear rationale as to why this work is vital and not just an 'add-on'. In some areas of the country, sexuality training is a mandatory element of induction programmes. This very positive step is one that FPA fully supports.

Training can help staff and carers work more effectively with ethical issues. It can build confidence in delivering proactive services via reflective practice and the development of specific practical skills. Ultimately, we expect that people with learning disabilities can feel empowered to make informed choices about what having a positive sexuality means for them. This could be helpful in building and maintaining a range of relationships and friendships for people with learning disabilities which could in turn enrich many aspects of their lives.

Useful resources

Resources from FPA

Contraceptive display kit
A briefcase style kit that includes samples of contraception and a male condom demonstrator.

All about us
This award-winning CD-ROM helps with the personal development and knowledge of people with learning disabilities around sex, sexuality and relationships.
For people with learning disabilities, their family carers and professionals.

Learning disabilities, sex and the law: a practical guide
Looks at legislation around sexual activity and people with learning disabilities. Includes capacity to consent, intimate care, record keeping and contraception. For front-line staff and professionals.

Out of the shadows: "Our voices aren't going to go quietly into the dark anymore."
Looks at the provision of relationships and sexuality education in Northern Ireland for young people and adults with learning disabilities.

Talking together about ... contraception
A two-book pack that supports young people with learning disabilities who wish to access contraception. For use by teachers and other professionals working with people with learning disabilities.

Talking together about ... growing up
Offers support to parents, carers and teachers of children with learning disabilities who are approaching or who are around the age of puberty.

Talking together about ... sex and relationships
A practical resource for schools and parents working with young people with learning disabilities.

To order FPA resources contact:
FPA
Email: fpadirect@fpa.org.uk
Fax: 0845 123 2349
www.fpa.org.uk
Tel: 0845 122 8600

Resources from other organisations

- www.bild.org.uk

Exploring sexual and social understanding
A knowledge assessment tool for adults with learning disabilities.

Sex and **Pregnancy and childbirth**
Accessible booklets for adults with learning disabilities.

- www.bodysense.org.uk

Desmond and Daisy
Anatomically correct male and female cloth models.

- ## www.changepeople.co.uk

Sex and relationships pack
Contains five easy-read booklets including *Sex and masturbation* and *Safe sex and contraception*.

- ## www.imageinaction.org

Let's do it and Let's plan it
Exercises and lesson plans for use with young people and adults with learning disabilities around sex and relationships.

- ## www.me-and-us.co.uk

Periods – a practical guide
Images and accessible text about periods.

Share special
SRE curriculum materials for young people with moderate or severe learning disabilities.

Sexual knowledge and behaviour
An assessment tool for use with young people with learning disabilities.

- ## www.pavpub.com

Becoming a woman
A teaching pack on menstruation for women with learning disabilities.

Sex and the 3Rs
An SRE pack for working with people with learning disabilities.

- ## www.rcpsych.ac.uk

Books beyond words
A series of books for people with learning disabilities including *Falling in love* and *Keeping healthy 'down below'*.

Useful organisations

How FPA can help you

Call **sexual health direct**, the helpline run by FPA. It provides:

- confidential information and advice and a wide range of booklets on individual methods of contraception, common sexually transmitted infections, pregnancy choices, abortion and planning a pregnancy

- details of contraception, sexual health and genitourinary medicine (GUM) clinics and sexual assault referral centres.

FPA helplines

England
helpline 0845 122 8690
9am to 6pm Monday to Friday

Northern Ireland
helpline 0845 122 8687
9am to 5pm Monday to Friday

www.fpa.org.uk
Visit the FPA website for confidential information and advice or send your enquiry to Ask WES, the FPA Web Enquiry Service at www.fpa.org.uk.

Ann Craft Trust
www.anncrafttrust.org
Works with staff to protect people with learning disabilities who may be at risk from abuse.

British Institute of Learning Disabilities
www.bild.org.uk
Provides information, publications, and training and consultancy services.

Change
www.changepeople.org.uk
A human rights organisation led by people with learning disabilities.

Image in Action
www.imageinaction.org
Works with young people and adults, publishes resources and provides training and consultancy around SRE for people with learning disabilities.

Mencap
www.mencap.org.uk
Works with people with a learning disability, their families and carers. Has a network of affiliated groups.

Norah Fry Research Centre
www.bristol.ac.uk/norahfry/
Evaluates and develops services for people with learning disabilities, including around sexual orientation and the client/staff relationship.

People First
www.peoplefirstltd.com
www.peoplefirst.org.uk (easy read)
An organisation run by and for people with learning disabilities to raise awareness of and campaign for the rights of people with learning disabilities.

Respond
www.respond.org.uk
Works with people with learning disabilities who have experienced abuse or trauma, or who have abused others.

Sex Education Forum
www.ncb.org.uk/sef
Information for professionals involved in SRE.

www.valuingpeople.gov.uk
Explains *Valuing people now* and how it is being put into practice for people with learning disabilities.

FPA supporting professionals

FPA membership

FPA members receive a range of benefits including:

- Discounts on FPA publications and resources.
- Discounts on FPA training courses.
- A quarterly enewsletter delivered to your inbox.
- An exclusive member-only area of our website.

Choose from three membership packages – Individual (£30 per year), School (£50 per year) or Organisation (£90 per year).

FPA training

As the leader in sexual health training in the UK, we offer high quality training that enhances skills to support people's sexual health and rights.

Our training is available in a range of options so you can choose what suits you best, whether it's on request, tailor made, consultancy or open courses. We also provide university accreditation for many of our courses so you can build up your CV or achieve credits by attending.

FPA publications and resources

FPA has a wide range of books, booklets, training manuals, CD-ROMs, DVDs and other resources on a variety of sexual health topics. Whether you're a health professional, teacher, learning disability professional, youth worker, researcher, parent, carer or policy maker, you will find a resource to help you.

For more details on membership, training or publications and resources see www.fpa.org.uk or call 020 7608 5240.